I Beat
DIABETES
You Can Too!

Also By Keithron Powell

It's Your Season Don't Miss It!

Preaching: Answering Questions Preachers Ask

How To Study The Bible From 5-1

How To Guide: Self Publishing

Trial of a Father and Son

Understanding Faith

Visit
www.kdpproductions.com

I Beat

DIABETES

You Can Too!

Keithron Powell

Special Thanks

I want to thank Dr. Anand Vakharia for diagnosing me but more importantly, for being upfront and honest. Thanks for not pulling punches and sugar coating the truth. Thanks for being in this business to save lives. I know that you are going to be moving on one day but I can say that you have been the best Primary Care Doctor I've ever had. You made a bad situation not so bad. Whatever you do... don't change. Your patients need you exactly the way you are.

I especially want to thank Gina Ernest RN, Certified Diabetes Educator and MY nutritionist. Thank you so much for taking time to explain in detail, diabetes, its complications and more importantly, how to eat properly. Because of you I gained the knowledge I needed to lower my blood sugar and my A1C. That information helped me come off of my medications and now I am able to help others. You truly saved my life.

I know doctors and nurses often don't get the reward, respect or the thanks they so rightly deserve. I know that often you don't see or hear from your patients until there is a problem or it's too late. I know most patients don't say thank you. On their behalf let me say...
Thank you for all you do.

I hope you both understand that I don't want to see you ever again and that's a good thing. (Smile) If I never see you at the office it means you both did your jobs but more importantly, it means I listened and did what you said. It means your advice was exactly what I needed to hear to make a positive change in my life. However, as bad as I don't want to see you two again, I truly hope that when I do visit the doctor's office, you two are there. Whether for a basic checkup or a serious issue, I hope I am coming to see you. You both showed that you care and that is what you want from your doctor.

I truly hope this show of gratitude reminds you everyday that you both are greatly appreciated.

Your patient... "Trouble"

Lastly, I want to thank my wife, Teresa. You have had to deal with this disease as much as I have, maybe more. Thanks for being my friend and for allowing me to sort through the many feelings I had, with patience and understanding.

I love you.

Table of Contents

Foreword

Introduction

Chapter 1   September 2013
             "You Have Diabetes"............................20

Chapter 2   What Is Diabetes?..............................27

Chapter 3   How Did This Happen To Me?...............35

Chapter 4   Insulin Is My Friend 40

Chapter 5   Change In Lifestyle.............................48

Chapter 6   Eating Healthy May Not
             Be Good For You................................56

Chapter 7   Measuring Your Food 69

Chapter 8   Discipline..78

Chapter 9   Myths & Misunderstandings..................89

Chapter 10   Don't Make Your Doctor
             Work Hard 102

Chapter 11   Watching Your Levels.........................112

Chapter 12   October 2014
             "One Year Later".............................118

Chapter 13   21 Day Challenge.............................127
             21 Day Chart 133
             Bibliography....................................135

Foreword

Keith Powell is man you would never forget. His talent doesn't stop with book writing. He also writes and plays music and, he is a preacher, a Man of God. I had the pleasure of meeting him, approximately one year ago. I wouldn't exactly say he was excited to see me, but, nonetheless, he sat with me, and he listened. I could sense that he was shocked and disappointed in himself, thinking that he could have been a better steward of his body. Nonetheless, he was an eager student. We chatted about many things, his likes, dislikes and how he could turn this ship around, to save it from running into an iceberg, called "diabetes."

Many of the people I encounter on a daily basis, are sent to me to learn how they can reverse or control the damage and destruction this disease brings with it. Surprisingly, they don't really want to be there. They don't want to hear words like, blindness, kidney failure, strokes, or heart disease. They want to sweep their little secret under the rug and keep living life exactly how they have been. They would prefer to pretend they don't have diabetes, and it will magically go away.

Each year, diabetes claims the lives of hundreds and thousands of people in the United States. It is the leading cause of blindness and kidney disease. It plays no favorites when it comes to race, religion or status. This disease will kill you if you let it. We all have illnesses, financial , and relationship problems. This book will take you on a journey that will draw on your emotions. Some of you will laugh, and say, "That's me."Others will cry and say, "I don't want this to be me." But I promise you, by the end of the last page, you will be inspired to make some changes in your own life, whether it is centered around diabetes, or some other challenge you may be facing.

That would be the first of many visits with Keithron. I taught him everything I could, to arm him for his battle. We spent many afternoons talking about his plans for the future, his music and his life. We became friends. He taught me as much as I taught him. He inspired me to not become complacent in my own life. His book is just one of the many gifts he has shared. This book is a must read. Take this journey. I promise you, you won't be disappointed.

Gina Ernest, RN
Certified Diabetes Educator

x

Introduction

Diabetes, disease, amputation, kidney failure, blindness and death. Those were the words that my doctor said to me that changed my life one day in September of 2013. Why? Because they were all directed at me and from that moment forward my life would never be the same. Never in my life had I heard those words directed at me in such a way that it seemed real. We've all, at one point or another, contemplated what or how we might die but to be given a series of potential outcomes that could become my reality was sobering to say the least. Do you want to live? That's the question every person with diabetes needs to be asked and that's what my doctor asked me.

The problem with being diagnosed with diabetes isn't just the reality of the disease but it's speaking with your doctor and realizing that you knew something was wrong before you entered the office and did nothing about it. You were wondering why you were so tired. You began to count the times

Diabetes is a silent and slow killer. It takes its time to destroy your body while you make excuses for the changes in your body.

that you had to go to the bathroom to urinate. You watched commercials, on TV and thought maybe you had some type of bladder problem. Then you justified your questions by saying you're only going to the bathroom because you're drinking a lot of fluids, not realizing or admitting that being as thirsty as you were is also unnatural.

Diabetes is a silent and slow killer. It takes its time to destroy your body while you make excuses for the changes in your body. The fact that you recognized the symptoms but ignored them can be irritating at best and frustrating at worse. You knew something wasn't right. You knew you didn't feel good. Yet, you did nothing about it and now your doctor is looking you in the face and saying words that are depressing and frightful.

Men are probably the worst. Most men despise going to the doctor so they'll do everything they can to NOT go. Most of which simply comes down to ignoring the problems they see in their bodies. Men will try to use the bathroom before leaving the house, like a toddler, or worse they'll plan their trips around the bathroom. However how do you justify that you can't sleep through the night without going to the bathroom three or four times?

The more questions the doctor asks, the more you realize that this is partly your fault. He asks, "Are you exercising?" and you say you don't have time. He asks, "If you've been gaining weight?" and all you can do is look at the bulge underneath your shirt and sheepishly say that you have. Or worse, you proudly say that you've miraculously lost weight without exercising. You've been bragging about your weight loss but what you don't understand is that it's a sign that you're truly sick.

There are few things you need to understand about this book. First, this book is not a daily account of my life beginning from my diagnosis but it is highlights of particular events, mile markers and memorials. I have recounted what I believe are the most important points over the past year of my life, each I believe, will be of benefit to you. Draw from my experiences, triumphs and even failures to better yourself. You don't have to die from this disease.

Second, this book, isn't a book to use as a self diagnosis. If you've received this book from a family member or friend and see yourself in this book DO NOT ATTEMPT TO FIX THE PROBLEM WITHOUT SEEING YOUR DOCTOR!

This book is for three people:

a) **The newly diagnosed**. If you have been diagnosed with diabetes, this book is going to help you to understand what's coming next and why you feel like you do. It will also help you to make a plan that you can execute to get better.

b) **The person that thinks they could possibly be diabetic and is seeking a diagnosis from**

a doctor. If you see yourself in these pages, GO TO THE DOCTOR and ask for a blood sugar test. It is best to know for sure than to think you're fixing the problem, by using this book and all you're doing, in reality, is making yourself sicker.

c) **The family member of a suspected or diagnosed patient.** The family of a diabetic patient needs to understand what's going on with their loved one as it affects you, as well. You also need to know how to respond to them, the diabetic, properly.

Next, this book is written in everyday language. I am candid and transparent. I want to make sure that you, my friend, understand what's going on in your body. I want you to hear the seriousness of this disease that shouldn't be overlooked or ignored. Because of this, I make some blunt statements, not for shock value but because they are true and real. However, the most important thing I want is for you to know that you don't have to die because of this disease nor from its many complications. You do not have to have a limb amputated. You do not have to worry about going blind or having kidney

15

failure. You can cut your chances of having a heart attack. You can turn your life around and beat this disease.

When the doctor and I sat in the office for our first real visit he explained the numbers I was seeing on the piece of paper he placed in front of me. He said my blood sugar level was 460. I remember when he first saw it, he looked puzzled and left the room. After a few minutes he returned and was relieved. When I asked why he said that he went to see if they needed to admit me to the hospital for further observation. Now, that was a shock to me because the last time I spent a night in a hospital was right after my birth. The worse thing I'd been to the hospital for since then was stitches from fighting and for broken bones from doing gymnastics. So, when he said that, I was taken aback.

He explained why that number, 460, was so serious and made sure I understood it. He then pointed to the A1C level which was 14. At first I didn't think it was a big deal until he explained. Afterwards, I was again floored. It was like being punched in the stomach. Here I was being told that those scary outcomes diabetes, amputation, blindness and even death were all possible realities for my future. The worst part was that I did it to myself. I was the one who didn't exercise. I was the one that stayed up late eating anything I wanted. No one forced me to do anything. This was my fault. Thats when I decided that if I got myself into this mess I was going to get myself out. I decided right

The irony of diabetes is that its tactics, strengths and weaknesses are all provided by you.

then and there that if diabetes wanted to bring those outcomes into my life it was gonna have to fight to do it. I wasn't going to go down easily. I was going to fight for my life.

That's what being a diabetic is. It's a fight for your life. You have to see diabetes as your opponent. The only way to win a fight against a formidable opponent, which diabetes is, is to understand its tactics and strengths, discover its weaknesses and counteract them. The irony of diabetes is that its tactics, strengths and weaknesses are all provided by you. Your weakness is its strength. To win against diabetes you have to overcome your weakness... you. If you don't, diabetes will win.

You are living with DIABETES but what you need to learn, is to LIVE with diabetes. You have to learn that you may not ever be fully freed from it because your body has a genetic predisposition for the disease but your actions can and will determine if the disease wins the battle for your life. You have to want to live more than diabetes wants you to not live.

The fight for life against diabetes is fought and then won or lost in the mind. You have to make a decision to live and then stick to that decision. You have to decide to live daily doing what it takes to beat this opponent. One thing you'll learn quickly is that you can't take a break in this fight because diabetes is fighting you daily, without a lunch break. Every morning, noon and night diabetes is looking for you to slip up so that it can do what it does best. It is relentless but you have to be even the more relentless.

This book is about fighting for your life against a disease that destroys lives and kills millions yearly. It's about not becoming a statistic. This book is about beating diabetes and you can. You don't have to be on medications all of your life. You don't have to stick yourself with needles for the rest of your days.

In this book you will read about how you can come off of medications but don't get the wrong idea. Not everyone reading this will come off of their medications. In fact, that shouldn't be your main purpose or goal. What you need to learn from this book is how to eat properly and healthy to live a full and long life, to slow the progression of the disease and avert its complications. The outcome of eating properly and doing everything your doctor tells you could be that you no longer have to take medications. Just be sure to not get discouraged if you don't come off of your medications. The purpose of this book is to regain some years on your life.

As you read my story, learn from it and put the things I mention into action. Discuss this book with your doctor and be sure that the things that worked for me are safe for you. My prayer is that you will read this book and turn you life around. My purpose in writing this book is to save someone's life. So, lets get started.

CHAPTER 1

September 2014
"You Have Diabetes"

In September of 2014, I was forced to the doctor's office. I finally, after about two years, was ready to admit that using the bathroom every two hours wasn't natural. However, this wasn't just because my wife had kept making a note to say that I spent way too much time in the bathroom, it was more than that. We had gone on a trip and were driving from Jacksonville, Florida to Atlanta, Georgia and I had the worst experience of my life. I had to stop every 1.5 to 2 hours and at one point I almost didn't make it. Talk about embarrassing.

It wasn't until I noticed I had absolutely no energy that I thought something has to be wrong with me. I was tired and sleepy all of the time and suddenly. I had a remedy for this unfortunate feeling. I drank a lot of juice. Now, by a lot I mean an inhumanly amount of punch, sweet tea and fruit juice. Anything with sugar in it was my friend. See, I discovered that I always felt better the more I drank. So, since I was always tired, sleepy and feeling horrible I drank more to feel better. Finally, my wife just said, "Babe, you need to go see a doctor." This time, instead of giving some sort of witty remark, like I usually would, I agreed.

After the doctor took my blood sugar he got a very unnerving look on his face. He paused and said, "I'll be right back," and left the room. When he returned he asked me easily, more than ten times how I felt. He began to explain that with a blood sugar level of 460, I shouldn't be feeling as good as I claimed. Honestly, I did feel fine. I wasn't tired anymore, not like I had been a month earlier. Prior the appointment I couldn't stay awake an entire day without a nap or two. By the time my appointment came I was back to "normal." He explained that he left to speak to another doctor about admitting me to the hospital because of my sugar levels. I was shocked because I was feeling normal. It wouldn't be for a few weeks that I would discover that my "normal" wasn't really all that normal.

The sentence that changed my entire life.

> *"Keith, you have diabetes."*

I will never forget that phone call. I was watching television when the phone rang. I answered and it was my doctor. After getting past the pleasantries he said, "I have some bad news." Now that is a statement that is never pleasant to hear but when a doctor says it, you really begin to think things over. He continued, "Keith, you have diabetes."and told me to come see him in the next few days.

When you first hear the word, diabetes, your response to it, while not exactly like everyone else, will have similarities. Typically, your response is based on your understanding of the word. This depends on your experience with the word and for many it is not a good one.

Some people have experienced the death of a loved one and as a result, are horrified of the very word, diabetes. Still others haven't had any experience with it and therefore they don't take it as seriously as they should. So, they don't do anything they are supposed to do as a diabetic. They eat whatever they want and they don't exercise. The two worse things you can do as a diabetic.

When my doctor and nutritionist spoke to me about diabetes they both said something that was very shocking, "No one has to die from this disease." I was puzzled by that comment because, most of the people I know, that talk about the disease, speak of it as a death sentence. So, to hear them say that, was a contradiction to my understanding. They explained that the problem was on two fronts:

a) **Diabetes is a silent killer.**
The thing that makes diabetes deadly is that its symptoms are not like most diseases. Diabetes symptoms, oftentimes, come on slowly and most people ignore the changes in their bodies. The increased frequency of urination and the onset of fatigue are often attributed to other things.

The sudden weight gain and subsequent loss, which should be a dead giveaway, are rather appreciated because, who wouldn't want to lose a couple of pounds?

b) Many patients lie.

Many diagnosed patients lie. They lie to themselves and their doctors about their eating habits. They lie about how they take their medication. They know full well that they aren't following the doctors instructions. Which is a lie that will be caught just as soon as the doctor does their blood work.

My doctor explained, "If you can just watch for the signs and symptoms and be honest with yourself about your diet, exercise and medication you can begin to get the disease under control." As I sat there listening to the doctor I made up in my mind that I wouldn't be a statistic. I wouldn't do what I had seen others do. For starters I wouldn't lie. I decided right there that I was going to beat this disease.

My doctor began to tell me about medications like Lantus, Metformin, Simvastatin and Lisinopril and how they worked. I asked my doctor a question, "How long will I be on medication?" You see, I am just like the average person I don't like pills or needles. I am not afraid of needles but I don't like them either. My doctor looked at me and with a very serious face said, "Keith, you'll be on some form of medication for the rest of your life." I looked at him in disbelief. That was just unacceptable for me. I couldn't believe what he was saying. I was a former athlete. I did gymnastics growing up and had even won several track meets for distance running. I couldn't accept that this man was telling me that I had to be on medication for the rest of my life.

> *"If you can just watch for the signs and symptoms and be honest with yourself about your diet, exercise and medication you can begin to get the disease under control."*

Without hesitation I said, "I'll be off all medication in one year." He immediately laughed and replied, "That won't happen." He explained how so many patients say they'll do right but always do whats wrong. He made it very clear that, based on his experience, there was no way I would do what was needed to be off of medication, especially in the time frame declared. I listened to him and simply said, "You'll see. I'm giving diabetes one year of my life."

You see, I like a challenge and for me this was yet another thing that I wasn't supposed to be able to do therefore it was nothing but another thing to concur. When I was a young boy my father, who was a boxer, began teaching me how to box. He taught me to not run from a fighter. He'd also throw a punches and teach me how to counter punch. He explained to me, that the counter punch was where you punished the guy for throwing a punch. If he throws one, regardless of if it lands, you hit him with two. Make him wish he'd never thrown a punch at all.

That is the attitude you must take with diabetes. You must see it as an opponent that can be overcome. You have to approach it daily like a prize fighter, knowing full well you'll be hit during the fight but recognizing that getting hit is only part of the process of you winning the fight. If diabetes throws one punch you counter that punch with two. You have to be vigilant in your stance and fight with this disease because it truly is a fight for your life.

CHAPTER 2

What Is Diabetes?

Ask any diabetic and their honest answer is that diabetes is a nuisance! It's an annoying disease that needs to be completely eradicated from the planet but lets get technical for just a moment.

Diabetes is a disease in which the person has high blood glucose (blood sugar), either because insulin production is inadequate, or because the body's cells do not respond properly to insulin, or both. This is very important to understand because it will determine what you need to do. Your illness must be diagnosed and understood before you attempt to control it.

There are 3 types of diabetes.

Type 1 Diabetes is where the body doesn't make any insulin and is often referred to as Juvenile Diabetes or Insulin Dependent Diabetes. People who suffer from this usually develop it before they are 40 years old usually as a child or teen. It is said to be the most rare as it only comprises about 10% of the diagnosed cases of diabetes. According to all research people who suffer from Type 1 Diabetes will have to take insulin for the rest of their lives because they do not make insulin on their own. It is the result of the pancreas' inability to make insulin leading to insulin deficiency.

Type 1 Diabetes is partially inherited, meaning that it is partially genetic. It can be triggered by a viral infection or diet. Unlike Type 2 Diabetes, Type 1 is typically, unrelated to lifestyle.

Type 2 Diabetes is when the body doesn't produce enough insulin or the cells don't react to the insulin the body produces. Approximately 90% of all diabetes cases are Type 2 Diabetes. Type 2 Diabetes can be controlled by losing weight, a change in diet, exercise and blood sugar monitoring. Type 2 Diabetes, however, gradually gets worse as it is a progressive disease. There is the possibility that a patient will eventually have to take some form of medication, usually in pill form.

If you are overweight you are at a higher risk of developing Type 2 Diabetes than someone that has a healthy body weight. People who have stomach fat or who are abdominally obese are especially at risk. If you lead a lifestyle of being physically inactive or eating the wrong foods you will contribute to the development of Type 2 Diabetes. Age is also a contributing factor as we get older typically because we become less active.

Gestational Diabetes affects women during pregnancy. Some develop high levels of glucose in their blood and their bodies are unable to produce enough insulin to transport it into their cells causing their blood sugar to rise. This can result in complications during pregnancy. Usually, this can be controlled with diet and exercise during pregnancy while some may have to take some from of medication. If the diagnosis isn't made the baby may be affected and become bigger than he/she should be.

Some people will be told by their doctor that they have **Pre-Diabetes**. This is where they have higher than normal blood sugar levels but not high enough to be considered diabetic. The body is losing its ability to produce insulin or is becoming insulin resistant. Your doctor will advise you to exercise and to change your diet. If precautions are not taken this will turn into Type 2 Diabetes.

Diabetes Symptoms
The most common symptoms are:
- frequent urination
- intense thirst and hunger
- weight gain
- unusual weight loss
- fatigue
- cuts and bruises that don't heal
- male sexual dysfunction
- numbness and tingling in hands and feet
- blurred vision (not specific to diabetes)
- headache (not specific to diabetes)

Complications
All forms of diabetes increase your risk for long term complications. The major long term

risk is damage to blood vessels. Diabetes also increases the risk of Cardiovascular Disease. About 75% of deaths in diabetic patients are due to Coronary Artery Disease.

Diabetic Retinopathy which is caused by damage to the blood vessels in the retina, brought on by increased sugar in the blood, which can result in gradual vision loss and potentially blindness.

Diabetic Nephropathy is damage to the kidneys and can lead to tissue scarring, urine protein loss and eventually chronic kidney disease, sometimes requiring dialysis or kidney transplant.

Diabetic Neuropathy is damage to the nerves and is the most common of all complications. The symptoms are numbness, tingling, pain and altered pain sensation which can lead to damed to the skin. Diabetic foot ulcers may occur and can result in amputation.

Additional complications include:
- Depression

- Hearing Loss
- Gum Disease
- Gastroparesis - the muscles in the stomach stop working properly.
- Ketoacidosis - the accumulation of ketone bodies and acidity in the blood.
- PAD (Peripheral Arterial Disease) - pain in the leg, tingling trouble walking.
- Stroke
- Infections

You need to know

You need to begin exercising ASAP but you more than likely have Ketones in your system.

- Ketones are substances that are made when the body breaks down fat for energy. In the case of a diabetic your body is making them but they aren't being used because you aren't properly processing your carbohydrates. As a result, your doctor will inform you that you need to exercise but that you may need to wait a period of time for the medication to get into your system. The doctor may not do a check because, it is assumed with diabetes patients that they have too many Ketones. The introduction of insulin medications will fix the problem. Consult your doctor.

- The Center for Disease Control and Prevention (CDC) says that 29.1 million people or 9.3% of the population have diabetes. Of that number 21 million people have been diagnosed leaving 8.1 million people that have not yet been diagnosed.
- Each year 12,000 to 24,000 people lose their sight because of diabetes. Diabetes is the leading cause of new blindness in people 20 to 74 years of age.
- Impotence affects approximately 13% of men and 8% of women who have Type 2 Diabetes. Approximately 50% to 60% of men over the age of 50 will experience impotence.
- Approximately 1 in every 400 kids and teens have diabetes.
- 215,000 people younger than 20 have diabetes.

All of these things are scary and true but you can do something about it to stall and even stop diabetes from affecting you in some of these drastic ways. Some things will not be reversible but you need to do what you can to educate and protect yourself from this point forward. Don't get discouraged, instead get angry and channel that energy into living!

CHAPTER 3

How Did This Happen To Me?

If you are normal, the first thing you're going to wonder is how did you get diabetes. You're going to listen to your doctor trying to explain to you what diabetes is and what it means and the entire time you're going to wonder, how did this happen to you. In fact, this thought will be all you walk away with after you leave your doctor if you aren't careful.

Even though I had made up in my mind to fight this disease, I still happen to be human and as a result, had to deal with the reality of the disease and this produced anger and depression. Both of these responses are normal. The question isn't if you will feel something. The question is how will you allow your feelings to affect you and your efforts. My decision to fight outweighed my anger and my depression.

My wife says that my attitude changed after my diagnosis and she was right. I became angry. I was angry with the disease but most of all I was angry with myself. I have always said that I never want to be my own problem. You see, I can understand when someone or something causes me to not reach a goal but to come to the understanding that it was my own efforts or lack of efforts, that prevented me from reaching a goal, has always been very upsetting. There is nothing more frustrating than being your own worst enemy.

> *There is nothing more frustrating than being your own worst enemy.*

The result of all of this was that I got angry and then depressed. I almost gave up. I almost said what's the use in trying. This was my fault and I deserved whatever I got. The odd thing was I didn't want people to know about my situation. I, unlike many people who will tell everyone about their illness, to gain sympathy, didn't want any sympathy. I wanted to this to be over and I didn't want to explain it to anyone.

I cut all my hair off. I told my wife I did it because my hair was thinning but that wasn't the full truth. I had been complaining about my thinning hair but this was a way for me to fight or punish myself. I took more pictures of myself at that moment than I've taken of myself in years. I was upset, depressed and angry. By cutting off my hair I was giving up. It was my way of protesting.

One day my wife was on the phone telling her sister about my situation and I overheard her and was livid. I instructed her to not tell another soul. I was so upset with her. I wanted to yell. I wanted to fight something, someone or anything. I was mean.

It took me a while to understand why I was so upset but I think it was because the disease was something I couldn't control while the secret was. For me, diabetes meant that I had lost control and I desperately wanted control again. As a result, with the exception of my church family, I told very few people.

Diabetes will affect you and your family. You have to be careful to not mistreat your family with your attitude change. Your family needs to learn to deal with their own depressions and fear of losing you. This disease affects everyone. So let's deal with the ugly truth about diabetes. You have it and it is partially your fault.

Now that we've admitted it, let's get past that and begin to fight! You got yourself into this mess and you can get yourself out of it. Make up your mind to stop this disease from ruining your life and the life of your loved ones. Make up in your mind that death is not an option. Get over your self loathing. Get over feeling sorry for yourself. Stop asking how did this happen to you. You know how it happened. Deal with it! Stop taking it out on everyone around you. It is not their fault.

Get over the fear of what could happen because while the truth could be bleak, it can also be glorious. It all depends on your next steps. What do you wan't to do? Do you want to live or die? If you want to die then do what you've been doing and diabetes will see to it that you get your desires but if you want to live, quit feeling sorry for yourself and do what it takes to live. Commit right now to a new way of living and watch your life change for the better. Its all up to you.

CHAPTER 4

Insulin Is My Friend

Diabetes is a progressive disease and you need to understand how this happened to you. First, you need to understand that it is partially your fault but also the fault of your genetic makeup. Eating sugary foods didn't do this too you, alone. You also, didn't catch it from someone like you do a cold. This is a disease, whose potential, was in you at birth. Add to that your bad habits and you have the perfect mixture for activating what's already in you.

This is why you need to understand it for your sake and the sake of your children. A good and healthy diet will go a long way to hindering your genetics from affecting you. It wasn't until I got my first injection of insulin that I understood how this disease operates in its progressive nature.

As my first examination progressed he began to explain to me that with my blood sugar and my A1C being as high as they were, there was no way that I could be feeling as fine as I claimed. That day he prescribed me insulin and explained how to use the needles. Once he was convinced I understood him he told me to not take it until I was about to go to sleep. I didn't ask why, I just agreed and was ready to leave. However, before I left he said, "You think you feel fine but once you take that insulin you'll feel differently."

That day I left and went to the drug store to get my medication. Like a good patient I read every line of the directions and warnings. I made the decision that I wouldn't stick the needles in my stomach rather I'd use my thigh. This turned out to be best as it didn't hurt as much. That night I was about to go to sleep and, as per the doctors instructions, filled the syringe with the insulin. Once I had taken the injection, I got into bed.

The next morning came and I awoke and something was different. I sat up on the edge of the bed almost immediately after my eyes opened. Unlike most every morning, for the past year or so, I wasn't tired but was fully awake. As I sat there pondering why I had all of this new found energy it dawned on me that I hadn't gotten up one time to use the bathroom. This startled me a little. I had slept and entire night and to my surprise, using the bathroom wasn't a necessity but an option. Yes, I had to go but for the first time in over a year it wasn't an emergency.

I sat there for a brief moment and then I smiled and reached for my phone. I called my wife and when she answered I said, "Teresa, insulin is my friend!" I felt like a kid learning to ride a bicycle for the first time and having that first success. I was a new man, well, maybe a renewed man. I no longer had to worry about getting sleep or sleeping longer to make up for what was lost. I could sleep like a baby without having to use the bathroom like one.

The next thing that was a welcomed shock was the fact that I had tremendous energy. I felt like I was 15 again. That's when I realized what my doctor meant by asking me how I felt. The truth is I felt fine but I didn't feel like I felt after taking that insulin. I felt bad by comparison the day before. The difference between how I felt sitting in that office, defending myself and how I felt sitting on the side of my bed that morning was light-years apart.

This caused me to realize that this disease gets progressively worse. It affects your organs and health overall but what you don't notice is that your body is adjusting to the bad feeling and it is becoming your new norm. It is like walking up a flight of stairs. Each step takes you higher and higher but unlike stairs this accent is bad for your health.

Your entire life is the first level where things are truly normal but at some point you begin to make the move to the next step. This is where you blood sugar is increasing because your pancreas is no longer functioning at its peak. Your A1C is beginning to rise. You may begin to feel a little "off" or you may notice that you're tired but it's normally just brushed off.

If you are a person that gets normal check ups your doctor may tell you that you are borderline diabetic. It is here that you are likely in the best place to completely stop diabetes because it hasn't actually done much damage. Unfortunately, many people do not get regular checkups and as a result they move up the stairs. More damage is done to their pancreas, they are probably gaining weight and they are beginning to use the bathroom even more but haven't noticed. They may even begin to notice that their vision is blurry but they are probably brushing it

> *Unfortunately, many people do not get regular checkups and as a result they move up the stairs.*

off as old age so they never go and get checked. They are even more tired but they just ignore it. Eventually, this feeling, that is not a good one, becomes the new norm.

This is how diabetes not only gradually gets worse but also how it gradually fools you into thinking that the way you feel is fine. By the time you realize that you don't feel fine you are in a bad state.

I was unable to run full speed for 50 yards. I had begun to have fainting spells when I did rigorous activities. I dodged the doctor by limiting my activity and learning to read the signs so that I wouldn't faint. As I moved further up the stairs, so to speak, at each level I'd feel worse but eventually I'd get accustomed to that feeling and accept it as my norm.

It would't be until August of 2013 that I would admit that I was sleeping way too much, tired way to often and that sudden and miraculous weigh loss couldn't have been normal. In fact, I was having problems believing that my wife's good cooking, without frying and using only fresh vegetables was truly enough to cause me to lose as much weight as I did. It wasn't until I took some full body pictures that I had to admit I looked like I was dying, even if no one else would admit it to me. The truth is I was dying. That's the day that the doctor explained to me what a diabetic coma was and that if I wasn't careful I could slip into one.

As I sat on the edge of my bed replaying my life and how I'd progressively begun to feel worse I felt a little fear at how well I was feeling after taking one shot of insulin. Exactly how bad off was I and how much damage had I done to myself by not going to the doctor? I wondered. I had climbed the stairs claiming to feel fine all the while getting sicker and this insulin didn't walk me down the stairs, rather it knocked me back down to what was truly normal. It was exhilarating and scary all at the same time. That was the second day that I knew I was going to make a drastic change to my life. There was no way I was going to go back to feeling like I felt before the insulin shot.

How did I get here?

I realized then the importance of going to the doctor even though you feel fine. Some sicknesses can fool you and your body can adjust to being sick and perform as if it's not. Not going to the doctor is a gamble I could no longer take. Of course there are people, who like me, didn't have insurance but you have to go and do something because your health is worth it.

How did I get here?

Well, I could blame the doctor I had over 10 years earlier in 2003 who, without checking my blood, diagnosed me as being borderline hypoglycemic and told me to watch my diet and to not eat greasy foods. It wasn't until I was sitting in the doctor's office being told all this information about diabetes, that my former doctor should have known that hypoglycemia is a symptom of diabetes. Imagine the look on my face when my doctor, who isn't black, said that whenever he sees certain symptoms in his black patients, that he immediately checks for diabetes just as a precaution and that my former doctor, a black woman, should have done the same or at least considered it.

Yes, I could blame her but the truth is my health is my responsibility. So, I do take some of the blame. I am the one who ate everything and anything I wanted. I am the one who stayed up late at night eating and going to sleep. I knew full well that I was gaining weight and made excuses to not exercise while pretending that I needed to gain weight. Somehow, I had convinced myself that this was a good thing. It's not like I didn't notice my stomach getting bigger. It's not like I didn't notice I had to buy an entire new wardrobe. That's how I got here. I did this to myself. I can't blame anyone but me and maybe my genetics.

CHAPTER 5

Change In Lifestyle

Now that you've dealt with the reality that you have this disease and have decided to fight it, you must also realize this isn't something that is going to end over night. Diabetes is a disease that happened over time and it is going to take time to get past it or to get it under control. So the first thing you have to do is learn how to live with the disease. This means a change in lifestyle in even in the most personal of areas.

The doctor explained to me that I needed to check my feet everyday to see if I was losing feeling. He explained that a loss of feeling could result in me needing some type of amputation.

This was a scary thought, to say the least. I had heard of people having to have toes and even feet removed as a result of diabetes and the thought of this happening to me was surreal. However, I reminded myself that fear was not reality. Fear is believing in the outcome of a thing even before the outcome happens. I chose to not have fear by believing in an opposite outcome. I chose to fight.

The doctor explained the importance of me not getting sick and that I needed to get flu shots every year. This for some is a non-starter but the truth is you NEED to take every precaution

Fear is believing in the outcome of a thing even before the outcome happens.

because so many things can add to the effects of diabetes. Sure, you may get sick as a result of the shot but the shot can protect you from the things that come to help diabetes fight against your efforts. A day or two of sickness, in order to be well, is worth it.

He also said that I need to have my eyes checked this wasn't something that I thought was that necessary until he said that diabetes can lead to blindness. I didn't want to go blind as a result of me being stubborn so, off to the optometrist I went. The good news was that no damage had been done to my eyes but the bad news was that I needed reading glasses. This didn't come as a surprise as I had noticed a change in my eyesight, even if didn't want to admit it.

Your eyes are the windows to your soul, as the saying goes but they are also a good place to see what's going on in your body. That blurred vision that you're experiencing may not be old age but it could be the result of high blood sugar.

Right after I was diagnosed I took immediate action to change my lifestyle. The doctor explained that my biggest problem was that I loved to drink fruit juices, punches and other items that were high in sugar. After hearing this, I decided they would be the first things I cut from my life. As a result, my blood sugar dropped from 460 on my first visit to 180 in ten days. I simply drank nothing but water with all of my meals and my body reacted to the change. That's the key, your body will respond to the change but you have to be serious about the change. You have to be disciplined.

When I went back to the doctor to pick up my glasses I no longer needed them. The eye doctor assured me that I needed them so, I told her to give me a test. She gave me something to read and told me how far away to hold it to read it. I read a portion at the distance she suggested, which I couldn't do before, then I moved it even close to my face and kept reading. Not only did my sugar drop but my eyesight cleared up from this simple change. The eye doctor said, "It looks like you wasted money on these huh?"

I had to learn to live with the disease but to not accept the disease. I accepted that I had the disease but I didn't accept what they disease wanted to do with my body. My body was mine and I decided that I would take control and responsibility over it. That's a major key in this fight.

Accept the fact that you have the disease but don't accept what the disease wants to do. Realize that acceptance leads to complacency and complacency leads to giving up and giving up leads to giving in. Giving in to the disease could mean amputation, blindness and even death and neither of those can be your option.

Why settle for death when there is a chance to not die?

I decided to live and to do so I had to not become a victim to the disease. A victim is someone that either can't fight or won't. The thing with diabetes is that most people can fight but won't. You have to decided daily to fight for your life.

Because diabetes is a slow and silent killer you must take every precaution concerning the disease. This means changing your lifestyle to combat the disease. One of the worst things you can do is get the attitude that says you don't care because we all die from something. That is not the mindset of a courageous person, rather it's the mindset of a person that is afraid and has given up on life. Diabetes doesn't have to win the battle for your life. Diabetes can be beaten!

What in your lifestyle led to this disease?
1) You probably have poor eating habits. You probably drink or eat a lot of foods that are high in carbohydrates (sugar).
2) You probably don't exercise. You, more than likely, are one that goes to work and sits all day and doesn't get much activity unless you

are on your way to the car or the refrigerator to get more sugary foods.

Here are a few things you will need to do daily to counteract and to monitor the results of diabetes. Every time you get into the shower slowly and methodically run your fingers across the bottom of your feet. Checking your feet daily is very important to monitoring your status. Also, apply lotion to your feet daily to keep them moist. Dry feet can result in cracks and sores. Sores, especially on the feet, are not good for a diabetic. Your doctor will perform a test at each visit. Do not lie to the doctor. If you don't feel something during the test admit it. A loss of feeling should be immediately reported to your doctor.

Pay close attention to your vision. If you notice a change, inform your doctor. Typically, a change in vision, especially blurred vision, is the result of high or low blood sugar. Either you've eaten too much or too little. In most cases, it is that you've eaten too much.

Notice when you are tired. Being tired all of the time is not normal. Excessive sleep is also not normal. Often, when your blood sugar is low, you'll become tired and lethargic this is either the result of not enough food or not enough exercise. You need to get moving. Your doctor will tell you to move at least 30 minutes a day and the first thing you're going to do is say, "I don't have time." However, you need to remember that if you don't make time to exercise you are making time to die.

The problem that most people have with exercise is thinking that they need to join a gym or buy expensive equipment. This is not the case at all. What you need to do is get moving. Go walking around your neighborhood. Go to a track and do a few laps. When I got back into working out I could barely walk 2 miles. Now, for me this was very disappointing because I used to run track and do gymnastics and now here I am getting winded walking. Now, I'm running a mile in under 10 minutes (9:35 is my fastest) and trying to get to 8 minutes.

You have to keep at it. You have to realize that it is going to take time to rebuild what you've let break down. Don't be discouraged by your inability to do what you did years ago. Start from today and do what you can and build on that.

The key to getting diabetes under control is to change your lifestyle and if you do you will begin to see a drastic change in your body and in your test results. You must take control or diabetes will. If you want to be free of medications and the fear of diabetes then you must take action immediately and daily.

CHAPTER 6

Eating Healthy May Not Be Good For You

Before I was diagnosed with diabetes, for breakfast, like clockwork, I'd have to have a peach and a plum with my bacon, eggs and toast (with jelly) and to wash it down I'd have either a large glass of orange juice or sweet tea. Throughout the day, I'd grab a couple more pieces of fruit and of course more sweet tea, punch or my personal favorite, orange juice. I remember thinking how good it felt to be eating so healthy because I didn't eat candy or cake when I wanted a snack but I'd grab a bag of grapes and dive right in. Because fruit is good for you…. Right?

As a diabetic, you need to learn that just because something is healthy doesn't mean it is good for you to indulge in. It turns out that I was doing all my damage with fruit, fruit juices, punch and sweet tea. I don't like pastas and breads that much so I don't eat lasagna, cakes and pies a lot. I am not a big candy eater at all. In fact if not for the occasional mint I'd almost never eat a piece of candy. So imagine my shock to discover that all the things I'd heard about how heathy fruit is, while true, didn't mean that it was okay to indulge. The biggest failure that diabetics have is thinking that just because it is healthy you can eat as much as you want. Fruit and fruit juices are a prime example. Yes, fruit is good for your body but for a diabetic it can be just as dangerous as drinking a bottle of soda.

Most of us know that fruit and fruit juice have what we call "natural" sugar but what we fail to realize is that sugar is sugar and it doesn't matter if it is "natural" or not because the body doesn't process any sugar properly, natural or otherwise.

The word carbohydrate is a fancy word for sugar. I was completely shocked when I discovered that fruits are all high in carbohydrates. As much as I love to eat grapes and by love I mean I can eat a pound or more in one sitting, I had to realize this was bad for me. So, they were removed from my diet along with all other fruits and fruit juices. I completely removed fruit from my diet for 10 days.

Now, I am not a big pasta or bread eater so by removing the main sources of my problem, fruit and fruit drinks, my blood sugar levels began to drop rapidly. It is key for you to recognize your biggest problems and remove them. For me, it was fruit, juice and punch and all other sugary drinks. For you it could be bread, pasta or some other food. Removing your biggest offender is only part of the battle. For others it may be a combination of things that you are eating that is causing you problems. You have to pay attention and be honest with yourself and remove what's causing you the problem. You must decrease all of your sugary intake to the levels that your doctor prescribes. If not you'll simply replace one sugary item for another.

The most shocking thing for me to realize was that food was my enemy, if I wasn't careful with it, even healthy foods. Fruits are good for a diabetic, in moderation. That is the word that every diabetic must remember, moderation.

The most difficult thing for a diabetic is to understand how to eat. Yes, there is a proper way to eat and this has to be learned, understood and practiced. If you don't get this right you will do even more damage to yourself and exacerbate your disease. This may seem harsh but too many carbohydrates are poison to a diabetic. At the same time carbohydrates are necessary to survive so you have to learn balance to eat carbohydrates in a way that isn't harmful to you.

The thing to do is learn the rules of your food. When a diabetic hears what the doctor says about their food and changing their eating habits, the only thing they hear is what they CAN'T have. So of course it seems like you can't get enough food to survive. You will look at the amount of food they suggest and think there is no way you are going to satisfied. This is far from accurate and only a trick that your mind plays on you. What you will learn, within about the first 30 days, is that there are other foods you can eat that will not have an affect on you at all. You will discover foods that you may have overlooked before, are now more pleasing. You will learn the importance of a snack and how to do it properly as well.

Typically, a diabetic is given between 45 - 60 grams per meal depending on your ability to control your diabetes. Now, the way it will be explained to you is that you will need to eat no more than 4 carbs at each meal. The very first thing you'll ask is which is correct? Do you get 4 carbs or 60 grams at each meal? The answer is both.

Here is how it works:

You're allowed 60 grams of carbohydrates or 4 carbs per meal. Every 15 grams equals 1 carb.

$$15 \text{ grams} = 1 \text{ carb}$$
$$15 \text{ grams} = 1 \text{ carb}$$
$$15 \text{ grams} = 1 \text{ carb}$$
$$\underline{+ \ 15 \text{ grams} = 1 \text{ carb}}$$
$$60 \text{ grams} = 4 \text{ carbs}$$

You should be eating 3 meals a day, minimally, so that you are eating 180 grams or 12 carbs per day. At first it will seem tedious and even a nuisance, with all the carb counting and food measuring, however, once you get it you'll be able to look at your food and have a good idea of the carb amount.

When you are buying food and preparing it you have to count the number of carbs in the food. We will cover this in a later chapter. The point of counting your carbohydrates is to manage your blood sugar levels. There are a few things every diabetic should be doing when they eat.

1) You should check your blood sugar before you eat. Knowing your blood sugar levels during your rest or fasting times is a good way to discover if your blood sugar is lowering. You can see if you're doing well with your new diet. It can also be a source of encouragement. So don't skip this first step before every meal.

2) You should count the carbs that are on your plate. You need to know what your body is doing with the carbs you eat. Your body has to process carbs but it needs a control. The amount set by your doctor will give you a controlled amount to discover what your body is doing with what you feed it.

3) Two hours after each meal you need to recheck your blood sugar. Two hours gives your body time to start processing the carbohydrates. As you perform these checks and record them, you will be able to see the progress your good diet is having or how your bad diet is failing you. By recording both the before and after levels, over time, you can see if your body is beginning to process the carbohydrates better.

When I eat breakfast now, I typically have 4 slices of bacon, three scrambled eggs with cheese, tomatoes, bell pepper, mushrooms and onion in them and some hash browns. With that breakfast I have only one food that has carbs in it, the hash browns. On the package of hash brown I eat one serving (ten pieces) which has 21 grams of carbohydrates. That's almost 2 of the allotted 4 carbs for that meal and for me that is enough. I don't have to have more carbs with my breakfast. If I wanted to, I probably could have some orange juice with that meal but I have chosen not to. So, I'll have the Walmart version of Crystal Light, because it's cheaper and because it has zero carbs and is still sweet.

I know what you're thinking. What about the cheese? Well, it turns out that the American cheese slices that I add to my eggs only have 2 grams of carbs per slice. If I add my 2 slices of cheese or 4 grams to my 21 grams from my potatoes I have only reached 25 grams for that meal or less than 2 carbs of my 4 carb allowance. Remember every 15 grams is equal to 1 carb. I didn't over indulge and I am full. Remember I am not a big carb eater but I guarantee the average person will be satisfied with that breakfast.

What happens when I go out for breakfast?

I love going to Cracker Barrel and like most people, I think they have some of the best biscuits around. Now, my wife and I don't go all of the time so this is like a treat. When I go I always order the Three Meat Breakfast. I modify the order to come with 3 sausage patties, 3 eggs over easy and of course the biscuits. I also add a side of hash brown casserole. So, how do I count the carbs?

Well, the meat and eggs are always 0 carbs, so they don't count. The hash brown casserole that they bring is the equivalent of about 30 grams or 2 carbs. I'll explain how I know that later. So, I'm half way there for that meal. The biscuits are where things get tricky. Typically, 1 biscuit is 1 carb so I know I can eat a maximum of 2 biscuits. Then I use either the sugar free jelly or the sugar free syrup. With this meal, that I eat, on special occasions, I've hit my carb allotment pretty much dead on and I've never walked away unsatisfied and wanting more to eat. Additionally, after eating and checking my blood sugar I've never spiked higher or even close to 120.

Buying Food

The first day of shopping after my diagnosis was a slow process. I walked into Walmart looking at every package, reading the Nutritional Fact Sheet and thinking, "This is going to be my lot in life." I felt like I'd be that old guy that I used to look at. You know the one with the cane, walking bent over who had 200 pill bottles at home and a timer to take them. As I walked the aisles I could hear my doctor say, "Stay out of the center aisles because thats where they hide the carbs." Because I had never had issues with carbs I had never really considered that the aisles were where the fattening foods were and the outsides was the healthy stuff but sure enough I began to notice it.

I immediately found myself looking at the Nutritional Facts on my foods and trying to see just how many carbohydrates were in everything I ate. As much as I hated to admit it, this was a necessary step if I wanted to not lose a limb or die. If I wanted to one day be off my medication and back to playing basketball or jogging, this was a necessary chore that I needed to hurry up and get used to. Looking at labels and counting my carbs had to become as natural as breathing. I had to see it as just as necessary also.

What happened?

As you make notes about your eating habits and blood sugar levels, you will see that your fasting (before you eat) levels are decreasing. This is a good thing but be careful that you are not starving yourself of carbs in order to get lower levels as this isn't healthy and could lead to low blood sugar or hypoglycemia. You must follow the diet plan as given as closely as possible. For me, it was easy to do because I am not a big carb eater. I typically eat less carbs naturally. My problem was the carbs I was drinking but your problem may be different from mine.

As you check your levels after your meals you will see some very interesting results. You will see your blood sugar has spiked. This is normal. Everyone has a spike in blood sugar after they eat even non-diabetics. This is because the system is being charged with glucose and is processing it for energy. The problem of the diabetic is that the pancreas isn't making enough insulin so the body can't process the sugar and as a result it is dumped into the blood increasing blood sugars levels.

Over time you want to see your spiking begin to drop. This is important as it means your body is doing better at processing carbs. It is also an indication that you are eating better for your body. Remember spikes are normal but the height of the spike tells you what's really going on in the body.

Your spikes, after eating, shouldn't be higher than 120. If you're consistently above 120 after a meal, and you've been doing what the doctor said concerning your carb intake and you're taking your medication properly speak with your doctor. Do not take the advice of a nonprofessional who tells you to increase your medication to lower your levels as this can be dangerous. You want to work with your doctor to cause your body to respond positively to treatment.

> *Do not take the advice of a nonprofessional who tells you to increase your medication to lower your levels as this can be dangerous.*

Remember that the goal is to come off the medication, if at all possible, or at the very least have it at the lowest levels. Typically, this depends on the amount of damage done prior to your diagnosis and on what you do after you've been diagnosed. Being diagnosed gives you the opportunity to take control over your body, your heath and ultimately your life. As with all diseases, early detection is always best. It can mean the difference between the damage being irreversible or not. However, early detection alone won't stop the disease from doing you harm. You must do your part to counteract the bad behavior that contributes to the sickness.

This is why you must go get your checkups and know your body. Don't be sick and pretend you're not.

CHAPTER 7

Measuring Your Food

When it comes to eating, the last thing you want do is have to pull out scales, measuring cups and spoons or some odd device to measure the amount of food you're eating. There are so many products and myths that it can be discouraging and this is why most diabetics give up and just eat what they want. Who has time for that? Well, in the beginning, you need to make time for it.

The key was what my nutritionist said to me. She explained that eventually, if I was diligent about learning how to measure my food, I'd be able to do it without any devices. So, for the first few weeks I paid very close attention to my portion sizes and over time I was able to look at the amount of food on my plate and determine if I could have more or needed less.

Measuring your food is vital to determining the state that your body is in. As stated in the previous chapter you are to eat no more than 60 grams or 4 carbs per meal. Measuring your food is how you calculate the carbs. If you want to slow the effects of diabetes you will have to do this.

Reading The Labels

One of the easiest ways to calculate your carbs per meal is to look at the package your food comes in. Today, unlike when our parents and grandparents were diagnosed, things are easier because all food is required to have the dietary chart on them. There are two sections you need to pay attention to; 1) Serving Size and 2) Total Carbohydrates.

The Serving Size and the Total Carbohydrates work together to tell you how this food will affect you and how much you can eat. Now that you know how many grams of carbohydrates are in a serving you can begin to measure your food portions. Remember that you are allowed 60 grams of carbohydrates per meal.

On this particular label you are shown that in 1 serving you will get 31 grams of carbohydrates.

Lets take this a bit further so that you can accurately count your carbohydrates. In the previous chapter I explained that every 15 grams of carbohydrates are considered 1 carb. You are allowed 4 carbs or 60 grams. So when you are adding up your carbs for that meal you need to be aware of what is on the label.

On this label you have 31 grams of carbohydrates or the equivalent of 2 carbs. This means you are half way to your 4 carb limit. To really understand how to count your carbs, by the numbers you must know that there is a system.

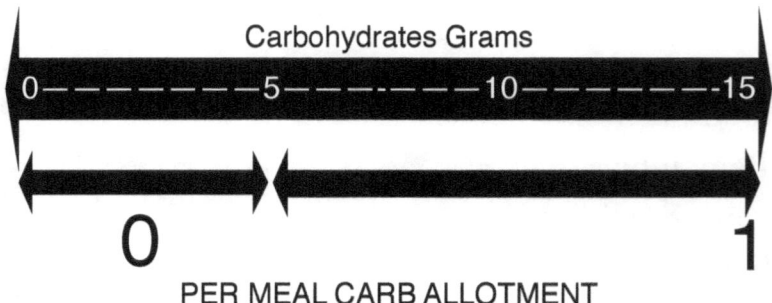

This chart shows you how to keep track of your carbohydrate grams so that you can count your carbs per meal. Any label that you read that shows the carbohydrates at 5 grams or less count as 0 carbs. However, don't be fooled into thinking that if you eat 5 things that are 5 grams or less that you are safe. Your grams do add up. So that if you eat 3 foods that are 5 grams each you have reached your 15 gram limit which equals 1 carb.

Once you go over 5 grams it is safe to begin seeing it as 1 carb. Just as with the carb adding below 5 grams you must keep track and add up the above 5 gram count until you reach 15 grams. This will keep you within your meal carb allotment.

Now would be a good time to look around your kitchen and see what foods are below 5 and what foods are above. You will notice that your meat items are all below 5 grams of carbohydrates. Most, if not all will say 0 grams. This means, technically, you can eat as much meat as you'd like without the fear of ever reaching 15 grams (1 carb). There are plenty of foods that do not have carbohydrates or that are below 5 grams. Please, however, listen to your doctor when it comes to eating anything that has 5 or less grams of carbohydrates. Do not assume that they are necessarily good for you. Over eating certain meats can be just as bad for your health eating foods with high carbohydrates.

It may seem, after looking at a few of the products in your refrigerator and pantry, that it is easy to go over and to not actually eat enough to be satisfied with your meal. This is why it is important to use your carbs wisely. If you are thinking of having pie for dessert you may want to cut back on some carbohydrates in the actual meal, to not go over your carb allotment.

Measuring By Sight

There are some specific guidelines for measuring your food when you eat. In the beginning you will become an expert on using measuring cups and spoons and while you are at home this is perfectly fine. However, what do you do when you go out to eat? Many diabetics make the mistake of eating too much when they are out at a restaurant. You have to have the discipline to say no to yourself and the understanding of how to properly measure your food.

When it comes to measuring your food what you are measuring is the foods that present the most danger, foods high in carbs. So, if you're eating a meal that has rice, for instance, you need to know that you can't have an entire bowl of rice if you are going to have some drink or other foods that have high carbohydrates. You have to remain within your meal allotment, even at a restaurant.

One easy way to measure your food is to use your hands. Remember your food carbohydrates are measured in grams but sometimes you can't count the grams so you need to use this system. 1 Serving = 1 Carb

Hand Portion	Serving Size	Food & Drink
One Fist	8 fluid ounces	Beverages
Two hands cupped	1 cup	Dry cereal, Stews, chili, Soup, Green salads
One hand (cupped)	1/2 cup	Rice, pasta, mashed potatoes, potato salad, fruit salad
Palm of Hand (typically a woman hand)	3 ounces	Cooked meat or fish
Two thumbs together (women's)	1 tablespoon	Salad dressing, sour cream, peanut butter, whipped topping
Tip of thumb (to the first knuckle)	1 teaspoon	Margarine, oil

This system will become easier over time and you won't actually have to put the food from the restaurant buffet on your hand to measure it. You'll be able to look at it and tell if that particular dish or item has too many carbs.

One of the issues I ran into wasn't in measuring the amounts but being able to eat enough so that I wasn't hungry after I ate the way all of the books and websites suggested. I quickly learned what foods to eat more of so that I wasn't hungry. In other words I learned that I could fill up on foods like salad, meat and other low carb foods without exceeding my carb per meal limit. Eventually, as you go to your favorite restaurants or even cook your own meals, you'll learn what you can and can't have as well as how much. This is going to be vital to you not messing up or quitting the routine altogether.

As with anything, at some point you are going to want to reward yourself for doing so well. You're going to say, "Hey I've been eating so disciplined that I deserve to be able to eat this or that." You'll even decide that it is fine to give yourself a day off from your diet. This is normal and encouraged, to a degree.

Taking one day or one meal every now and then to celebrate is not a bad thing however, be careful that you don't get into a habit of rewarding yourself, as harsh as that may sound. It is human nature to continue to make excuses for reasons to celebrate and before you know it, you're eating wrong 4 days out of the week. When you reward yourself, you are adding all sorts of things to your diet that you know you don't need. Don't fall for the "reward myself" trick. Remain disciplined because your life depends on it.

CHAPTER 8

Discipline

The truth about the human body and the world we live in is that they were designed to work together. Our problem is that most of what we do works against our bodies. Don't think that I'm going on a rant about global warming, no, rather I'm speaking about how we treat our bodies because of how we treat and eat our food. There seems to be a natural drawing to things that aren't really good for us. We like sweets and food high in carbohydrates because they taste better. However, as we've all heard growing up too much of a good thing can be bad for you.

Diabetes is a fight between the body and the food you feed it. Your body is telling you there is a problem with your diet. When most people think of diet they immediately think of losing weight but when you're diabetic it gets a little more complicated than simple weight loss. In short, you are killing yourself with food. Most people won't see it this way but it is like eating poison. A very slow acting poison; whose

How do you not question that you're going to the bathroom every two hours?

symptoms and even the outcome are, in most cases almost unnoticeable, until it's too late.

The statement, "almost" unnoticeable, is key because a diabetic really does notice the changes in their body and habits. The problem is ignoring them. How do you not question that you're going to the bathroom every two hours? How do you not question the lack of energy, tiredness and your inability to stay awake? How do you not question that you're gaining weight or losing it rapidly without exercise? In fact, diabetics will experience weight loss and if they are not careful, they will appreciate the weight loss and not acknowledge what it really means.

What about the fact that you can't run 40 yards without feeling like you've run ten miles? Those signs that you keep ignoring will lead to nothing but heartache and can, ultimately and unfortunately, lead to death. This however is the reality that most people don't want to admit and as a result a great many people lose limbs and/or die as a result. Diabetes is a killer that doesn't have to kill. It warns you of a problem and provides you with time to correct it and yet people still die from it. So, why do people experience the worst when it comes to diabetes? Simply, in most cases, it's their diet.

When you are diagnosed with diabetes you are assigned a nutritionist, at least you should be, and they are supposed to show you a video to educate you on diabetes and your diet. The problem with this video, in my opinion, is that it is too benign and after watching it, I can see why people don't take this disease as seriously as they should. Of course, I do understand why the video is so PG-13 as to not scare people but the truth is it probably should be a little bit more graphic and show the real possibilities of this disease, in all its gory detail.

Discipline

After watching the video and speaking with my nutritionist I asked, "Can you please talk to me direct and tell me the worst case scenario?" She paused and said, "Keith, you could die from this if you don't do what's right." That statement carried so much weight but it didn't scare me. What it did was brought a sobering reality to my situation. I didn't see diabetes as a death sentence, rather I heard the second part of her statement loud and clear, "...if you don't do what's right." This put things into perspective for me. It let me know that my life was in my own hands and not the disease's.

As she and I began to discuss the video and the disease more, she explained that most people have to have amputations or die, not because the disease does anything but because they won't do what they need to do to prevent its complications and she said it all starts with diet. Your diet is the key to whether or not you live or die from the complications of the disease. I realized right away that diet can only work if I was disciplined.

After hearing my nutritionist, I began to think about every diabetic I had ever known and how they treated food. I even had the perfect example of what not to do in front of me, a married couple who were both diabetics. Often we'd go to breakfast and they'd both order 2 or 3 pancakes and a tall glass of orange juice along with all the regular breakfast staples. I'd begin counting their carbs but not telling them what I was doing. They'd always be over the carb count limit.

Once, they began discussing with me how they approach eating their food, their explanation of carb counting, was completely in error from what I'd read and had been taught. Of course, they said that their doctor had told them their blood sugar levels and eating habits were fine. The problem was that I noticed they were constantly complaining of being tire. They both stayed ill in some way or another and all of their symptoms were those of diabetes.

I often wondered how they could claim to be fine if they were repeatedly ill. After years of dealing with the disease they were both still on medications. I wondered why the material I was reading from my doctor and online, was completely different from what they were saying their doctor told them. I couldn't understand why I was getting better, by that I mean having my medication dosage lowered, while they were constantly sick, back and forth to the hospital and not having their medications decreased.

Each time I'd go to the doctor I'd discuss what I was seeing and hearing from them with my doctor. The couple had been attempting to give me advice on the disease because they'd been dealing with it for some years now. They wanted to make sure I understood the disease however, the more I listened to them, talked with my doctor and remembered what I'd seen from other diabetics, the clearer the problem became to me. When it comes to food, the biggest problem of diabetics is their inability to deny themselves the pleasures of certain foods.

Many of us have strong cravings for many different types of foods. However, when you are suffering from this disease, your cravings and desires can be deadly in the long run. This is why I say the video that diabetics are shown and even the way the doctors speak to their patients need to be more graphic and honest. You have to decide if that cake or pie is worth dying for. When you look at your love of pasta, ask is it worth dying for? When you see that cola or that doughnut is it really worth dying for?

Keeping your diet comes down to discipline and that hinges on your will to live. At each meal you must ask yourself if you really want to live or not. You can't act like it's fine to take a break from your sugary boycott. You have to the conclusion that sugar is killing you. Your body can't take it anymore and you must realize this is a real dilemma. As a diabetic you must learn that you can't live to eat but you must eat to live.

When I sit at the table to eat, even now, I am counting my carbs. I keep reminding myself that food can be bad for me, if I'm not careful. This is a lesson that all diabetics need to learn, remember and respond accordingly. You have to remember that you are sick and don't let the medicine fool you into thinking you aren't.

When you are placed on insulin your body responds almost immediately and that response feels great. For the first time in years you have energy. You feel like you can run a marathon. You will feel like your old self again but that feeling can be misleading.

Many diabetics make the mistake of thinking that because their medicine makes them feel better they can eat anything. Do not fall for the trick of thinking that your medicine makes it perfectly fine to eat all you want, like so many people do. Your medicine isn't counteracting your bad habit. You are doing even more damage to yourself by doing this.

Your medicine is not designed to be a bridge or enabler. It is designed to make you better but it isn't able to do this if you're not using it properly. All you're doing is making your body more and more dependent on the medication. Your body stops wanting the food and now craves the medication.

You must realize that food is not only the reason that you became a diabetic but it is also the main reason you remain diabetic. So, if you want to reverse that truth then food will be the main reason you do so. Your approach to food will determine your entire life dealing with this disease. When I visited the doctor for my diagnosis they immediately thought I was eating cakes and pies but it was the fruit and juices that were killing me. You have to admit what's killing you.

Diabetes makes all carbohydrates bad, even the ones found in fruit. I had to learn what you have to learn, that I must deny myself of the thing I like most. Denial doesn't mean you can't have it but it does mean you have to watch how much you have. You can eat fruit and you can even have sweet tea but the question is, do you have the will power to not overindulge.

For some this may seem extreme but I immediately cut all of my fruit and fruit juices out of my diet. Neither my nutritionist nor my primary care doctor could believe how fast my blood sugar levels had dropped nor that I had made such a drastic change to my diet. Why? Because most people won't do what is necessary to change. When they asked me why I made such a drastic change I replied simply, "I want to live." That's the attitude you have to take. Are you willing to do what it takes to live? Sure, potato chips are good but life is better.

Diet isn't about starving yourself nor is it all about denying yourself. What it's really about is limiting yourself and being honest about those limits. That takes discipline. Every diabetic is different and yet the same. We all have to be honest with our limitations which are pretty much the same. For this reason we all have to count our carbs, take our medication as directed, check our blood sugar and not cheat on our diets. We have to be disciplined.

Another food I love is cheese cake and normally when a cheese cake is in my presence I can't help but eat it. However, I am a diabetic so normal for me, can't be normal anymore. I was given a slice of cheese cake back in January of 2014 and it took me three days to eat one slice. For some this may seem unrealistic but it shouldn't. For a diabetic a slice of cheese cake can be a bad thing. I can of

However, I am a diabetic so normal for me, can't be normal anymore.

course have cheese cake, just like anyone else but I can't eat it like everyone else. I have to be mindful of the fact that my body can't handle it, because it can't. I am sick and so are you. Even when we don't feel like it. We have a disease and the first line of defense against diabetes is our diet.

On one visit, my doctor asked how I as doing so well and I explained that I have to take this disease seriously and be disciplined because I am the only one that can make the change. The same is true for you. Your diet brings on the symptoms but its up to you to admit that the symptoms are really signs of a deeper issue. You have to decide to have discipline so that your diet doesn't kill you.

CHAPTER 9

Myths & Misunderstandings

It was the first Thanksgiving after being diagnosed and we were in Dallas, Texas with some family. The smell of the food filled the air and I was looking at it and thinking of how I couldn't wait to eat. There was candied yams, turkey & dressing, sweet potato pie, cheese cake, ham, collard greens and more and my eyes were wide open because all of my favorites were on display. I'm sure I was openly licking my lips. Someone saw me looking at the macaroni and cheese and said, "You're diabetic, you can't have that." It was at that time I remembered what my nutritionist told my wife during our consultation.

She explained that there were some myths and misunderstandings about diabetes concerning what people with diabetes can or can't eat. She also said the worst thing you can do to a diabetic patient is dictate or police what they eat for them. She explained that when you do this, you frustrate them because they have a hard enough time trying to deal with the disease and most people place more boundaries on them than necessary. The simple truth is most people don't fully understand the disease.

In the beginning, even after the nutritionist explained this to my wife and I, my wife still had issues with my eating habits. "You can't have that!" she'd say in protest of my food choices. She was trying to be helpful but all I heard was someone telling me what to do. This didn't start an argument but it was just as frustrating as the doctor said it would be. I would always say, "Baby, you've got to learn what I am learning about the disease." Most of what people believe about diabetes is based on myths and misunderstandings.

The "You Can't Eat That" Myth

When a diabetic is told what they can't do it comes across, to them as a personal attack. They are already dealing with the reality of the disease, disappointment about the disease and even fear of the disease so, the last thing they need is to be told they are doing yet again, something else wrong. Diabetes plays with the mind of the patient and by telling them what they can't have you only do more damage to them mentally.

Most people believe that you can't have cake, pie or even fruit juice but this is not the case at all. A diabetic can eat anything they want. The issue is understanding the definition of moderation and portion control.

Every diabetic must first understand how to measure their food. For many, this event takes away from the joy of eating but again you must ask is this cake worth dying for? Of course it's not. If you want to eat cake then you must learn portion control. You must be disciplined in your eating. Just because you can have it, doesn't mean you can have that much of it. It is here that most diabetics fail.

You're accustomed to eating as much as you want. You've practiced this all of your life but unfortunately, you're a diabetic and as such, you can't do exactly what you like. You have to remember that it is a matter of life and death.

> *According to the American Diabetes Association, diabetes causes more deaths each year than breast cancer and AIDS combined.*

No one wants to be treated like a child and if this is the case, then you've got to handle your food like an adult. Take responsibility for yourself and your food. Eat what you want BUT stick to the rules concerning your food. You can't have an entire slice of pie if you've already eaten your carb allotment for that meal.

The "Diabetes Isn't A Serious Disease" Myth

The truth is that if you manage your diabetes properly you can prevent or delay diabetes complications but don't let that lull you into a false sense of security. According to the American Diabetes Association, diabetes causes more deaths each year than breast cancer and

Myths & Misunderstandings

AIDS combined. Two out of three people with diabetes die from heart disease or stroke.

The "If You Are Overweight or Obese, You Will Develop Diabetes" Myth

Being overweight is a risk factor but family history, ethnicity and age are also contributors. Many people assume, wrongly, that weight is THE risk factor so they overlook the others. According to the American Diabetes Association, most overweight people never develop Type 2 Diabetes and many of the people with Type 2 Diabetes are normal to moderately overweight.

The "People With Diabetes Must Eat Diabetic Food" Myth

This is completely untrue, in fact, the diet that a diabetic should adhere to, for the most part, is the same for anyone who wants to have a healthy diet.

The "I Feel Better" Myth

Many diabetics do themselves the most harm when they feel better. They will purposefully change their diets and begin to eat anything they want for two reasons:

1) The doctor said they can eat anything they want (which is not the entirely true) and;
2) Their medicine is making them feel better.

The only reason you're feeling better is because you've been taking medication and not because you're cured. The truth is, even if you were given permission by your doctor to stop taking medication, you're still a diabetic. You can't switch your diet back to what got you sick in the first place, just because you feel better. Diabetes is always in you. Don't feed it (no pun intended). Don't give diabetes what it needs to do you harm.

The "If you have Type 2 Diabetes and your doctor says you need insulin it means you're not eating properly" Myth

The truth about diabetes is that it is progressive. Over time it may be determined that your diet or your oral medications aren't capable of keeping your blood sugar low. Your doctor will then prescribe insulin because your body has totally ceased to make enough on its own. Don't be discouraged, using insulin to keep your blood sugar levels low is a good thing and it works.

The "Medicine Counteracts" Myth

What many diabetics do is take their medication, especially insulin, just before or right after they eat what they know they shouldn't have eaten. This is very irresponsible and dangerous for the diabetic. Do not make this a habit. In fact, this behavior is proof that you have not understood your medication and what its there to do.

Your medication is supposed to help you process sugar but that doesn't mean you can eat anything because of what it does. Your doctor has prescribed you medication and

The goal of your doctor is a healthy you, not necessarily, a medicine-dependent you.

he's also told you how to diet with the hopes that you will heed his warning so that you might get better. Your doctors goal is to, in so many words, reset your body. He wants you to be off of the medication, if at all possible. This is why they talk about possibility of lowering your medication. The goal of your doctor is a healthy you, not necessarily, a medicine-dependent you.

You will never get off your medication, which is what you should want to do if possible, if you're treating your medication like it cancels out your bad habits or gives you a free pass to eat improperly. Your medication is not a permission slip to cheat on your diet. Speak with your doctor and you'll discover they wan't to cut your dependence on your medication. All you're doing, by eating horribly and then taking you medicine to counteract the food, is prolonging your dependence on the medication and possibly further damage to your body. You'll never be free of needles and pills if you continue to commit this act. You're feeling better but your aren't completely better. Don't do something to set yourself back.

The "Diabetic Family" Misunderstanding

This disease is a dilemma for the diabetic family. Yes, it is a diabetic family because, it takes everyone working together to help the diabetic stay on course but your family can't help if they don't understand the disease. You can't explain it to them if you don't understand it either.

If you have diabetes, your family has diabetes (in a manner of speaking) and needs to be educated on it. This is the only way to not suffer from the frustrations of their misinformed help. Your nutritionist should schedule a meeting with you and your loved ones to educate you all on the disease because your family will have questions about it just like you.

What's worse than misinformed support is for a diabetic to have no support at all from family members. Most often, family members of diabetic patients, don't realize that they are contributing to the delinquency of the patient. They, because of their ignorance about the disease, do everything wrong, often unwittingly, to cause the patient to have setbacks.

I was speaking to a young lady about her father who is a diabetic. She said that when he was living in the nursing home, his nurses were very good about the food that he ate and as a result he had been pulled off his medication. However, since he had moved in with her, he was back on his medications and she didn't know why. As we spoke more she complained saying, "He doesn't eat right." she said explained further, "He eats what he wants to eat." I asked her "Who is buying and cooking the food for your father." She answered, "I am." I asked her if she bought food for him that he could eat or prepared it specifically for him. She said, "I do the shopping and the cooking."

One of the most challenging situations for a diabetic is not always in what they eat but what the family buys and cooks for them. It is in the home that most people do the most damage to themselves or have the most damage done to them, by the very ones that love them. The family of a diabetic has to understand that this disease is one that may require help from the people closest to them. If a person was a drug addict, the family would attempt to shield them from all others that use drugs so that they won't relapse. This is the same attitude the family of a diabetic should have. The family needs to help protect them from what can hurt them.

It is in the home that most people do the most damage to themselves or have the most damage done to them, by the very ones that love them.

There is a thin line between protecting and smothering so the family must be careful. The easiest way to do this is to remember that the diet of a diabetes patient is the same that every person should eat to remain healthy, with a few additions and limitations. So, if the family makes the changes, not just for the patient but for themselves also, everything becomes natural and easy.

Can the family do what's right for the patients survival? The truth is most diabetics do wrong simply because the family hasn't made the adjustment to help them do right. It is easy to tell them to do right but do you love them enough to help them do right?

It is easy to tell them to do right but do you love them enough to help them do right?

When I was speaking to the lady about how her father was eating and she told me that she did the shopping and the cooking, I asked why wouldn't she buy foods that were beneficial of him. She paused when I asked that question. She had been placing the blame on him when she was the one in charge of what came in the house. She didn't realize that he wasn't eating wrong because he wanted to but her, elderly father, was no longer being given a choice to eat healthy.

I said to her, "I don't know if you know this but you're killing your father." She couldn't believe what I had just said but that was the truth she needed to hear. She said she'd never thought about it like that. I asked her, "Would you give your father cyanide to drink?" She looked at me with utter disbelief and I continued, "That's what sugar is to a diabetic. It is poison if not eaten in moderation."

The diabetic and his family have to control what they eat. If this is not taken as seriously as it needs to be, the diabetic and their family will inevitably suffer the consequences.

The question is would the family rather deal with a little grumbling over new food choices or helping someone whose blind, can't walk without assistance because they've lost a limb or worse, attend a funeral? All this simply because the family couldn't make better food choices in the grocery store.

One of the first things we did in our home, after my diagnosis, was to get rid of the sugar in my home. Thats' correct. We don't have regular sugar in my home. My wife uses Truvia and I use the Walmart version of Splenda and I haven't missed sugar yet. I have programmed myself to see sugar as a poison. It may sound extreme but it keeps me on my toes and aware of what goes into my body. If you're a diabetic or the family member of one, please think about it exactly like that.

CHAPTER 10

Don't Make Your Doctor Work Hard

I remember going to one of my appointments and the doctor asked, before they took my blood, "Have you been eating right and taking your medication?" Without a thought I said, "Yes, I have." My doctor looked at me and said something that I hadn't considered, "If you're lying I will know because your blood work never lies." This is when he explained the myth about medicine that so may believe. He told me no matter what, if I was not being honest it would show up in the tests. The fact is, that if you're eating properly and taking your medication your blood sugar should come down which means your A1C should drop. It's simple logic. If you're not feeding yourself ungodly amounts of sugar then it can't be in your system.

Your doctor is frustrated because you are fighting his efforts to save your life. He can only tell you what to do, you have to do it.

After he got my tests back he was ecstatic because my sugar was not only remaining lower on my tests but because my A1C had begun to come down. That's when he sat down across from me, in the examination room and explained what many doctors may never admit to their patients.

Most patients frustrate their doctors by lying. If your doctor truly wants whats best for you he is going to get upset when he realizes you've been lying. We often think that they are frustrated and mean simply because they are overbearing, ego driven control freaks but that's not it at all.

Your doctor is frustrated because you are fighting his efforts to save your life. He can only tell you what to do, you have to do it. He's doing his job and so should you. He's diagnosed the disease, prescribed the medicine and the diet and all he wants you to do is, do what you're supposed to do to survive. He is not your enemy at your checkups. He's on your team and you're fighting him by NOT doing what he said and then you're lying as if he won't know. He may not say he's frustrated but trust me he is because, he knows your lies can cause you to lose limbs or worse, kill you.

Many doctors are blamed for not doing their jobs but why should they take the blame when you won't do what you're supposed to do to survive? This is your life and your words are saying you want to live but your choices, the thing that actually matters, are saying you want to commit diabetic suicide. Do you really think your doctor wants to cut off your foot? Do you really think he wants to get the news that you've died? Many people use the excuse that the doctor only wants to make money off of them by prescribing unnecessary medications or by doing

> *Many doctors are blamed for not doing their jobs but why should they take the blame when you won't do what you're supposed to do to survive?*

unnecessary surgeries but the truth really is, that most patients do not do as instructed so these doctors have no choice.

My doctor sat across from me and spilled his heart about his frustration with his other patients and I appreciated it. It showed me that I wasn't a meal ticket and that he was in this line of work to save lives but more importantly it showed me that if I was beaten by this disease it was nobody's fault but my own. I had to continue doing what I was doing. I had to take my medication daily and eat like I wanted to live.

I had already made up in my mind, on my very first visit, that I was gonna beat this disease but when he opened up and told me what he was really thinking on my second visit, I knew I had to do what was right. I had to stay on the track I was on. No cheating! No missing my medication and of course, check my blood sugar!

Your Blood Sugar Log Booklet

When you get your blood sugar monitor you will also receive a blood sugar log booklet, unless you get a monitor that is completely automated. Either way, you need to keep good records. It may seem like a nuisance to you but this will help the doctor get a picture of what your body is doing with your carbohydrates and it will help you to know when you've made a mistake in your diet.

Keeping a physical log is best. The physical log helps you keep track of the actual food you've eaten in addiction to your blood sugar levels. Your log booklet is a window into your past that will help you make corrections to your diet that will shape your future. If you know what you've eaten you can see if it is bad or not.

Do you need to remove something from your diet? Is it safe for you to add something to your diet? Your notes of your blood sugar levels and what you've been eating will tell you what you need to know so that you and your doctor can make the right decision about your heath.

This is also your doctor's quickest tool before checking your blood. If you've been honest and precise in your record keeping, your doctor can look at your notes and make determinations about your medication. Should it be increased or lowered? Can you go from insulin to Metformin? All this can be discovered in your notes. Make your life and your doctor's easy by doing what you're supposed to do.

You will quickly discover that the blood sugar log booklet that comes with your blood sugar monitor isn't very large so, its difficult to keep track of everything you've eaten. It is best to create a separate one for your food. You will discover that keeping a record of the food you've eaten will be invaluable.

You should check your blood sugar before you eat and again 2 hours after you've eaten. At first this may seem a bit much, with all the poking of your fingers but its is well worth it. Your booklet is not just a record so that your doctor can see what you've been doing but it is your daily tool as well. Often, when you're spiking really high, its because you've eaten too much of something or because something had more sugar than you expected. By keeping track and watching your levels you can, at a glance, see what's bothering you and what's not.

This is also a good place to keep track of how what you've eaten affects you, including your medication. Did you get sick after taking your medicine? Are you experiencing diarrhea or constipation? These are questions your doctor is going to ask you and keeping records is key to your treatment plan.

One evening we went out to a restaurant. I had been keeping good records and I had been watching what I was eating. At dinner I ordered a Philly Steak and Cheese sandwich and it of course came with fries. Now, I hadn't had a pretty high reading in a while. So, I ate the sandwich and the fries. My plan was to only eat a few of the fries but since I hadn't had a high reading in a while, just like you, I went for it. I ate the entire plate of fries.

Later that night I checked my blood sugar and guess what? It was high. I was so disappointed in myself. I learned a valuable lesson and I tried, with all that was in me, to never do that again. I thought about it very hard and realized I probably would have been fine with the sandwich and a few fries but not the entire plate of fries.

The record of what I was eating became my friend. Whenever I spiked very high I immediately asked myself, "What did I eat?" By keeping constant track of my food I was able to control spiking and eventually I developed a habit of staying out of the "too high spike zone." This not only made me happy but it made my doctors life easier. Because of my policing of my food and my records, my doctor could make informed decisions about my medication. As a result my insulin amount began to be decreased by my second doctor's visit.

Make your life the life of your doctor easy by being honest with your results, your food intake and by always bring your meter and notes to your appointments. This will be key in you moving towards coming off of your medication.

One last thing I learned from my doctor was that many doctors give up on their patients. This may seem cruel but it's the fault of the patient. Every doctor wants to save lives but most have patients who lie or just don't care and do the very thing they've been instructed to not do. Others are guilty of mistrust of doctors because they've heard stories about bad doctors and they take their fear out on their doctor.

Many doctors become somewhat jaded and insensitive, not because they are mean but as a protection for themselves. They've grown weary of losing patients, especially, after providing them with the information that could've saved their lives. Their attitude is a coping mechanism because losing a patient hurts. I believe that, for many, they simply find it easier to assume that you are not going to do right to make it easier to deal with the bad news they are going to have to deliver to you in the end. As a result of years of disappointment, they become detached and desensitized. This isn't a good thing but it seems to make sense.

That's what I felt from my nutritionist. She, really didn't believe I would do right and her surprise was evident at each visit. She told me a story about one patient who was getting worse at each visit but she swore she was doing everything she was supposed to do. After getting caught in her lies, on the tests, the lady finally admitted that she wasn't eating properly. The look on my nutritionist's face while retelling this story to me was one of concern, disbelief and disgust.

She explained that she was waiting to hear the bad news that this woman was suffering some complication as a result of her not adhering to the doctor's advice. The nutritionist was visibly affected by this patient that wouldn't do right and she said that a large percentage of her patients weren't doing right. After hearing that, I made sure that I came to visit her and give her my results at every appointment. If she wasn't there or couldn't see me because she was with another patient I left a message or sent her a text on her cell phone. She is the one that made me really understand diabetes. I refused to be another bad example for her. She had enough of those. I wanted her to tell a different story about me.

After one of my visits with her she said, "I really wish you could come and talk to my other patients because maybe you can reach them as a patient where I can't as a doctor." I really wanted to do it and she said she was going to check into it. My primary doctor also said the same thing to me after one of my visits but more than likely, there was some bureaucracy that prevented it.

You need to keep accurate records not just for you but for your doctor. Help your doctor by not being a source of frustration. Become your doctor's great example and source of inspiration.

CHAPTER 11

Watching Your Levels

The most difficult thing for me was to get an understanding of what was a good level and what was a bad level. To me, anything in triple digits was bad. If my blood sugar level was 86 prior to eating and then 110 afterwards, I was upset. I never wanted to see a number more than 99. My doctor explained I was being too hard on myself and that I was safe as long as my after meal number was not above 120. This was liberating.

Taking control of your numbers is as simple as watching what you eat at each meal. Remember, you are allowed 60 grams or 4 carbs at each meal. When you look at this individually you will discover that 1 carb or 15 grams isn't a lot depending on where it is coming from. So, you have to be strategic in how you get your carbs.

Many people fail at maintaining a proper diet, as a diabetic, because they feel they can't eat enough to get full. The key then is to find out what you can eat more of to replace what you can't have a lot of. I removed all fruit juice from my diet and replaced it with Crystal Light. By doing so I still got the satisfaction of drinking a fruit drink but I had absolutely no carbs. This meant that I didn't have to count my drink in my meal allotment and I could even have that second glass. Once I learned that meat had no bearing on diabetes I knew I could eat as much as I wanted (with limitations). So, my two favorite things were covered.

What you can't do is completely cut out your carbohydrates because they give you energy and you need that. If I was eating a sandwich I quickly learned that a bun was typically 2 carbs or that two slices of bread was about 2 carbs. That meant that a sandwich took up half of my meal allotment. Just remember though, I could stuff that sandwich with all sorts of meat and vegetables and feel satisfied. So where do I spend my carbs? Well, maybe a couple of cookies or a small bag of chips it just depends on the dietary chart of the product to determine what's good for me.

The key was learning to eat more of what didn't count and less of what did, while meeting or coming in lower than my carb allotment. This lowered my levels. This works fast and has some other benefits as well. By lowering my carbs, I began to lose weight because I was eating more salads and other healthy foods.

Here are some things to remember about your numbers:

1) A low number is bad but not necessarily a problem. Low numbers mean you don't have enough sugar but it depends on how low they are. My doctor never seemed to have an issue with my blood sugar levels reading about 77 or so during my fasting periods (early morning mostly) from time to time. There would've been and issue, however, if I would've been dropping into the 60s or less, consistently. This is why you can't completely remove the carbs from your diet. You need

them. At the same time high blood sugar readings 2 hours, after a meal, that is below 120 is not a bad thing.

2) Your food directly contributes to your levels. The goal is to develop a habit of eating foods that keep your levels within normal parameters.

3) The numbers don't lie. If your numbers are too high or too low check your food. If you can honestly say that you've been eating properly and your records show it, your doctor will be able to determine if you need to increase or decrease your medication. This is why you have to be honest. If you've removed all the carbs from your diet your numbers may drop too low and your doctor may lower your medication, assuming the medication is the problem. This can be disastrous. You must eat your carbs so that your body responds naturally, your doctor can properly regulate your medication so that you can begin to get better.

If you're not honest and you've been eating a lot of carbohydrates but fudging your records, your doctor may increase you medication to levels that they don't have to be all because you won't do what it takes to control your levels.

There are two people who can have an effect on your blood sugar levels, you and your doctor. You are primarily responsible because your daily choices have the biggest bearing. Your doctor can only respond to what you are doing. Most of the time, doctors are attempting to counteract the bad decisions of their patients while their patients blame the doctor for them not getting better.

It is not your doctor's fault if you don't do what the doctor told you to do. The doctor didn't give you that piece of pie that you knew you shouldn't have eaten. The doctor didn't force you to eat those two plates of spaghetti with those three slices of garlic bread. You did that on your own. Your doctor isn't trying to make money off of you by upping your medication or giving your two more types of medications. Your doctor is reacting to what

> *There are two people who can have an effect on your blood sugar levels, you and your doctor.*

you're doing to your body and trying to prevent you from doing yourself more damage.

One thing I learned about my doctor was that, while he was always cheerful at seeing me, he didn't want to see me. He longed for the day that I didn't have to come see him and there is a safe bet that your doctor feels the same way. The key to not seeing your doctor is to take control of your blood sugar levels.

CHAPTER 12

October 2014
"One Year Later"

Each person that reads this book is at a different stage of the disease. As a result of my diagnosis, I was able to do exactly what I said I would do, come off medication in one year. That doesn't mean that I may never have to go back on my medications. I understand what you need to as well, that there is a possibility that I may never take another pill or use another needle in my life time. That possibility gets better as long as I do what I am supposed to do. As a result, I don't take my food lightly. I examine everything I eat. I still count my carbs at every meal and every snack. Because, although I am not on medication, I am still a diabetic.

When I was on my medication I would get upset if I missed a dosage. I was so hard on myself. I was very serious about confronting and defeating this disease and I was gonna fight with everything I had. The reason that I was so adamant was because everyone I knew that had the disease had complications and I refused to be like them. I've seen people that have lost limbs or that are always sick and in the emergency room and I refused to be like them because the doctor told me that I didn't have to be like them.

The biggest kick in the pants was to hear my doctor and my nutritionist say that they didn't believe I would do right because none of their other patients ever did right. That made me want to be the one they always spoke of in a positive light. I wanted to be a different kind of example.

Just over one year later I went in for my final visit. My doctor came in and had the reading from my previous blood work. He opened the door and as he always does said, "Keith, my man!" I was nervous because in every visit I would make mention that at the end of one year I'd be off of medication. This visit was that one year visit and even though I had gotten good news at every visit, I wondered would I get even better news today.

My most memorable appointment, up to that point, was the time they removed me from insulin and placed me on Metformin. When he consulted with his boss they agreed that the decision to take me off of insulin was a good idea. I was ecstatic, although I tried to hide it. When I came out of the exam room, there were a few nurses and some doctors standing outside waiting to see me. They looked at me amazed and one said, "Congratulations." The main doctor asked what I did to get off of insulin within about 6 months and I simply replied, "I did what my doctor said."

That transition, from insulin to Metformin, was exciting and scary all at the same time. There was part of me that wondered if my body would respond favorably to this new drug. There was another part of me that still quietly held the fear that maybe I wouldn't be able to get off that drug.

Over the months of taking Metformin I began to notice that after some time, I'd get sick. I'd have diarrhea. It took me a moment to figure it out but as time progressed my system would begin rejecting the medication. Each time I went to the doctor he'd lower the medication and I'd feel better. At each visit I'd always mention that I was coming off the medication soon and his lowering the dosage was proof. When we finally got down to about 500mg my doctor said, "If all goes well you may be off by the end of summer." That made me excited and put us right at the one year mark.

Now, one year later, I'm sitting in the office and I've been waiting to see what the chart is going to read. When he gave me his usual high five and sat down he asked the normal questions but said nothing about the chart. As the exam went on he finally asked, "So, what did you think about your A1C?" I was totally confused because I hadn't been told what it was.

At my previous visit it was 6.5 and I explained that I didn't know what it was since then. Turns out they never sent me anything in the mail like they normally do and he didn't realize that. He got exited and said, "You don't know?" he continued, "Keith, your A1c is 5.7." Now, I knew that was low but exactly how low I didn't know. I had been shooting for a 5 but that seemed difficult to reach, so hearing 5.7 was a bit of a shock. He then said, "Keith, technically speaking, if this had been your very first visit, I'd be telling you that you are pre-diabetic." That was a shock to my ears. I just froze for a moment and he said, "Keith, technically, you can't claim to be a diabetic anymore." That blew my mind.

I had been working very hard to watch my diet. I had started jogging and lifting weights. I had been very disciplined and hard on myself after doing everything wrong for years and here is my doctor telling me I had done everything right. I had succeeded. My A1C was 5.7 down from 14, in one year. My blood sugar was also down to normal levels. I felt great, really great. Now the weight of diabetes had been lifted... well, sort of.

I looked at him and he said, "I think we can take you off of your medication." That was the statement I'd been waiting to hear. That was my goal! That was what I had said I was going to do at the very first visit.

He starred at the charts on the computer and said that there was no real reason to keep me on medication but that he needed to go and speak with his boss. That's when he said he was going to go fight for me. See, the truth was, according to my doctor, what I had done was not the norm so getting his boss to agree to taking a diabetic patient off of their medication wasn't going to be easy. He grabbed my paperwork, stood to leave and said, "Wish me luck."

As he left the room I got a little quiet. Being a pastor you'd think that I'd start praying right away but I didn't. I was a little nervous so I grabbed my phone and turned on the radio. After about a minute I said a simple prayer, "Lord, thank you."

The doctor stayed gone longer than I had expected. As the time passed I grew more nervous. I tried to be a "man of faith" as they say at church but this was unnerving. The longer he waited the more my mind ran. "Maybe he won't let me off." I thought. I tried everything I could think of to calm my nerves but nothing truly helped. Suddenly the door opened and startled me. The doctor exclaimed, "Congratulations! You're off of your medication." I was so relieved.

I couldn't believe it. I had done it. It was finally not a dream or a confession but it was reality.

We sat down, after another high five, and talked about what this meant. He said that his boss wasn't going to agree until she realized I was the guy that had been doing so good all year. They decided to give me a chance. He began to explain that they wanted to see how I did for 3 months and that I still needed to check my blood sugar levels. I didn't care what they said I had to do. All I cared about was that they said I was off of those medications. I'd done this much so I'd do whatever they asked of me.

> *I also took note that he didn't say I wasn't a diabetic. I am still a diabetic who is diet controlled verses insulin or medication dependent.*

I also took note that he didn't say I wasn't a diabetic. I am still a diabetic who is diet controlled verses insulin or medication dependent. Because of this I can't stop what I've started. I have to continue to measure my food and count my carbs. Each year I still need to get my eyes checked, get my flu shots and of course go in for all exams.

Just as diligently and disciplined as I was when I was first diagnosed, I must continue to be so. The progression of diabetes can't be cured but I can keep it at bay. I can take control of my life. Most importantly I can live my life and so can you.

From this day forward, take control of your life. Live it to the fullest. Don't take for granted your family, friends and even your enemies. Go outside more to watch a sunrise or to just stare at the stars. Read that book you've been saying you were going to read. Whatever you do, live.

Don't let diabetes be the reason you're depressed. Don't allow it to steal your life or your joy. You have the disease but don't let it have you. You control it and don't let it control you. This is your life, your body and this is all about choice. Choose to live.

Set small goals and keep track of them. Be harder on yourself than your doctor or family is on you. Don't get complacent. Don't accept your fate. Don't give up! Don't feel sorry for yourself rather be encouraged that you can still do something about it. Don't allow depression to tell you that life isn't worth living because that definitely isn't true. Look at your family and know they will not be better off without you. As long as you have breath in your body you have time and a chance. The saying is that it's not over until the fat lady starts singing. Well, I don't care how bad it looks don't let her get to the microphone.

Today is a new day and tomorrow hasn't come, yet. You can define your tomorrow today by living today, not like there is no tomorrow but like you have things that you ARE going to do tomorrow. You don't have time to die. You have your child's football game to attend. You have your daughters wedding to attend. You have that dinner planned with your spouse, at your favorite restaurant and you've made the reservations. Your anniversary is coming!

I beat diabetes and so can you.

CHAPTER 13

21 Day Challenge

By now you are pretty well educated in most things diabetic. It's now time to put this knowledge into practice. However, for many this will be the hardest part. So let's simplify some things.

When you meet with your nutritionist they are going to show you a video then give you some documentation. This documentation can be a bit overwhelming and even confusing. It is going to look like they are asking you to become a mathematician while suggesting that you barely eat enough food to satisfy a toddler. This typically results in many diabetics giving up on the doctor's orders and quickly reverting to what was doing them harm in the first place.

For me it wasn't as bad but don't take that to mean it was easy. I had to make up in my mind that I was going to live and to do so I had to first get a clear understanding of the disease and secondly, actively change my life. If knowing is half the battle, as they say, doing has to be the other half.

The nutritionist showed me a list of foods that I needed to stop eating or not eat so much of. The problem was, that I wasn't eating those things. I had an altogether different problem. The way I dealt with my diabetes was to immediately cut out the main source of my problems, the drinks. While it is probably safe to say that your eating habits aren't the best, because most of us don't eat well, as a diabetic you've developed a love for sugary drinks. You're probably buying juices by the carton and filling your refrigerator up with them. You're probably going through them in a matter of days. This is a result of the diabetes causing your body to crave liquids. This needs to be stopped.

First, your doctor is going to give you medication, probably insulin and you will immediately lose your thirst. However, a loss of thirst doesn't mean that you can drink less and do your body any good. You need to remove the sugary drinks from your diet. This includes but is not limited to: soda, fruit juice, fruit punch, sweet tea, Gator Aid (and like drinks) and sugary alcoholic drinks. This may seem a bit extreme but diabetes is also extreme.

If you remove the sugary drinks and replace them with either water or a Crystal Light drinks and diet drinks your body will begin to heal. The good news about this switch, I discovered, was that my family couldn't tell a difference in the taste. So that meant that it was easy for me to switch and my wife still got her sweet drink fix, only healthier.

We don't always realize it but our drinks are usually the most sugar filled portions of our meals. If you recall I explained that my blood sugar dropped from 460 to 180 in 10 days. During that time I drank nothing but water.

Next is to cut down on carbohydrates (sugar) from other sources. If you're used to having 4 and 5 pancakes with breakfast, stop.

Have only 2 and don't make them the size of the skillet to make up for not having more. Remember, the key is to replace them with things that you can eat that don't have an adverse affect on your health. Change your syrup and jelly to sugar free. You will not notice a difference in the taste in the syrup and you may notice a slight difference in the texture and taste of the jelly.

Remove all fruit from your diet. This was pretty difficult for me because I love grapes, plums and peaches. However, this was a change I needed to make. As a result I haven't had grapes in over a year. I miss them but I realize that they are very high in sugar. Now, I do understand that I can have a few grapes, however, I have chosen to just not have them and make other food choices that are not just healthy but safe.

If you are a pasta, bread or potato lover either cut down or remove them for 21 days. By doing just these few things you will notice a drastic drop in your blood sugar readings. When the 21 days are over and you've looked at your readings, don't make the mistake of thinking, "I'm done so let me go and eat all the stuff I removed." Rather, look at the progress you've made and ask is it worth it to set yourself back? Hopefully, you'll do this for the first 21 days, see the results and then continue for another 21 days. If you do this between your doctor visits you should see a drop not only in your blood sugar levels but also in your A1C.

It is your A1C that the doctor looks at to see if your medication should be increased, decreased or ultimately stopped. Also, by doing this, your doctor can get a clear understanding of where your body is and how much damage has or hasn't been done to it. The good news is that if you do this properly, you'll discover what foods affect you most and you'll learn if you can add certain foods back to your diet, in moderation, of course.

The first time I saw my doctor he was scared and spoke to me with a somber tone. After I did this simple plan that I've outlined thus far and continued doing it. My doctor would come into the examination room and give me high fives. He started calling me, "The man with the plan."

Compliments are encouraging and compliments from your doctor are the most encouraging of all because they mean you're getting healthier. Don't expect a compliment from your doctor if you haven't been doing what you were supposed to be doing. Take the 21 day challenge and watch your doctor give you compliments. Use the chart at the back of this book to record your results.

If you'd like more details concerning the number of carbs in certain types of foods or need clarity on carb visit the links below. Please see the Bibliography for more helpful links.

https://www.bd.com/resource.aspx?IDX=9850

https://www.bd.com/us/diabetes/docs/portion-control.pdf

21 Day Challenge Chart

Log your blood sugar readings for the day

| Date | Breakfast | | Lunch | | Dinner | |
	Before	After	Before	After	Before	After

21 Day Challenge Food Log

Food	Breakfast	Lunch	Dinner	Notes

Bibliography

Chapter 2 What Is Diabetes?

What is Diabetes?
http://www.diabetes.org/?loc=logo
http://en.wikipedia.org/wiki/Diabetes_mellitus

Definition of diabetes types.
http://www.medicalnewstoday.com/info/diabetes/
http://en.wikipedia.org/wiki/Diabetes_mellitus

What causes diabetes?
http://www.medicalnewstoday.com/info/diabetes/
http://en.wikipedia.org/wiki/Diabetes_mellitus

Complications of Diabetes
http://www.pamf.org/diabetes/whatis/

Diabetes Statistics
http://www.pamf.org/diabetes/whatis/
http://www.medicalnewstoday.com/info/diabetes/

Keytones:
http://www.webmd.com/diabetes/ketones-14241
http://en.wikipedia.org/wiki/Diabetes_mellitus

Myths & Misunderstandings
http://www.diabetes.org/diabetes-basics/myths/
http://www.medicalnewstoday.com/info/diabetes/

Center For Disease Control (CDC)
www.cdc.gov

Chapter 6 Eating Healthy May Not Be Good For You
How it works
https://www.bd.com/resource.aspx?IDX=9850

Chapter 7 Measuring Your Food
https://www.bd.com/us/diabetes/docs/portion-control.pdf
https://www.bd.com/resource.aspx?IDX=9850

Carbohydrate To Carb Count Chart made from speaking with nutritionist.

Hand measurements
https://www.bd.com/us/diabetes/docs/portion-control.pdf

Chapter 9 Myths & Misunderstandings
http://www.diabetes.org/diabetes-basics/myths/
http://www.medicalnewstoday.com/info/diabetes/

Did this book help you?

Keith would love to hear from you.

Contact Keithron Powell:

kpowell@kdpproductions.com
www.kdpproductions.com